Master Your Hunger: A Guide to Mindful. Eating and Conquering Cravings"

Master Your Hunger:
A Guide to Mindful Eating and Conquering Cravings"
By
Dr. Duane R. Hernandez

Title page

Table of Contents

Disclaimer

Master Your Hunger: A Guide to Mindful Eating and Conquering Cravings is intended to provide general information and guidance on mindful eating practices and strategies for managing cravings. The content within this book is not intended to be a substitute for professional medical advice, diagnosis, or treatment. Readers should consult with a qualified healthcare professional before making any significant changes to their diet or lifestyle, especially if they have any underlying medical conditions or concerns.

The author and publisher of this book make no representations or warranties regarding the accuracy, completeness, or suitability of the information provided. The reader acknowledges that they are solely responsible for any decisions they make regarding their health and well-being based on the information contained within this book. Furthermore, the strategies and techniques outlined in this book may not be suitable for everyone. Individual results may vary, and success in mindful eating and conquering cravings is not guaranteed.

By reading this book, the reader agrees to release the author and publisher from any liability for any loss, injury, or damage incurred as a result of following the advice or recommendations presented herein. Thank you for your understanding and for choosing to embark on this journey towards mindful eating and greater well-being with Master Your Hunger.

Description

"Master Your Hunger: A Guide to Mindful Eating and Conquering Cravings" offers a transformative journey towards a healthier relationship with food. In this insightful guide, (Dr. Duane R. Hernandez) unveils the power of mindfulness in overcoming cravings and mastering hunger. Through practical tips, mindful eating exercises, and personalized strategies, readers will discover how to tune into their body's cues, navigate emotional triggers, and cultivate a balanced approach to nourishment. Whether you're seeking to shed unwanted pounds, break free from restrictive diets, or simply reconnect with your body's wisdom, this book provides the roadmap to reclaiming control over your eating habits and fostering lasting wellness. Embrace mindfulness, conquer cravings, and embark on a fulfilling journey towards a healthier, happier you with "Master Your Hunger."

Introduction

Do you ever feel like you're trapped in a cycle of poor eating habits? Constantly grabbing for sugary snacks, mindlessly devouring full bags of chips, and then promising to start over tomorrow, only to slip back into the same pattern? You are not alone. Our modern society bombards us with tempting, calorie-laden goodies, and it's easy to get caught up in a wave of mindless eating. But what if there was a way to break out of this loop, unlearn harmful eating habits, and regain control of your health?

Breaking the Bite Cycle is your guide to mindful eating and a better relationship with food. Avoid fad diets and rigorous regimes. This book digs deeper into the science of mindful eating, assisting you in identifying your specific triggers for unhealthy choices and providing you with practical tools for developing healthy coping mechanisms. It has nothing to do with limitation, but with acknowledging your consumption practices and acquiring durable alternatives that suit your

Breaking The Bite Cycle: Unlearn bad eating habits and reclaim your health.

Do you ever feel like you're trapped in a cycle of poor eating habits?

Constantly grabbing for sugary snacks, mindlessly devouring full bags of chips, and then promising to start over tomorrow, only to slip back into the same pattern? You are not alone.

Our modern society bombards us with tempting, calorie-laden goodies, and it's easy to get caught up in a wave of mindless eating. But what if there was a way to break out of this loop, unlearn harmful eating habits, and regain control of your health?

Breaking the Bite Cycle is your guide to mindful eating and a better relationship with food. Avoid fad diets and rigorous regimes. This book digs deeper into the science of mindful eating, assisting you in identifying your specific triggers for unhealthy choices and providing you with practical tools for developing healthy coping mechanisms. It's not about restriction; it's about knowing your eating habits and making long-term changes to fit your lifestyle.

Imagine:

Beginning the day feeling energized and focused, powered by nutritious choices.

Say goodbye to afternoon slumps and cravings with smart snacking habits.

Approaching meals with presence and pleasure, appreciating every bite.

Being confident in your ability to make healthy decisions, especially in difficult conditions.

Breaking the Bite Cycle is the key to unlocking a healthier, happier you. Are you ready to give up the guilt and embrace mindful eating? Let's go on this trip together and reinvent your relationship with food, one delicious, mindful mouthful at a time.

Part 1: Recognizing Your Consumption Patterns

Chapter 1: The Reasons Behind Our Diets

Habits' Power

Bad habits are impossible to completely break. Strong habits mean that your brain will constantly be looking for the reward when the trigger presents itself. You can, however, change up the routine. The routine can change, but the cue and reward must remain the same.

We refer to this as the Golden Rule. Treatments for alcoholism, obsessive-compulsive disorder, and hundreds of other harmful behaviors have benefited from this rule.

Any negative habit can be broken. But figuring out the cue and the reward is crucial. Next, figure out a fresh regimen that will yield a similar outcome.

For instance, you might smoke as a means of social interaction or as a quick fix for excitement. You can get some coffee in the afternoon if you need stimulation.

Making this easy adjustment will improve your chances of effectively quitting smoking.

Changing your beliefs is a crucial component of breaking unhealthy habits and is likely the most significant one. Though the exact mechanism of action is unknown, research indicates that one needs to have faith in the possibility of transformation to bring about long-lasting change. For instance, you must first believe in yourself if you want to stop smoking—that you can break the unhealthy habit.

Beliefs typically only come into being with the support of a group. Find a support group or someone you can talk to about it every day if you want to break a habit.

Recognizing Your Cues in Food

Have you ever thought about how many choices we make every day about food and eating? We are constantly exposed to environmental stimuli, also known as external eating cues, which can affect our food choices and portions.

For example, portion sizes can affect how much food we think is proper to eat, and eating while preoccupied can affect how much food we eat overall.

Unlike external eating cues, our bodies have internal cues like hunger and fullness signals that can help us consume the right foods in the right amounts.

When they feel satisfied or no longer feel hungry, those who follow their internal cues quit eating.

As we age, a multitude of external variables impact our eating habits, perhaps leading to a disconnection from our internal cues. The phrase "eating disinhibition" describes this detachment from our bodies' requirements, which can lead to eating for reasons other than hunger, eating to cope with uncomfortable emotions, or consistently eating past fullness.

They might also alter their eating habits, such as cutting back on their intake if they intend to have dessert.

Identifying Your Body's Cues to Eat

The idea of being intuitive when it comes to following your body's cues on when to eat or stop eating. It has been demonstrated that utilizing cues linked to hunger and fullness is somewhat associated with reduced symptoms of disordered eating, increased body positivity, improved self-esteem, and maintaining a healthy weight.

Being open about one's cravings

Knowing your hunger cues will also make it easier for you to distinguish between physical hunger and cravings, which are frequently associated with emotional hunger.

It has been demonstrated that utilizing cues linked to hunger and fullness is somewhat associated with reduced symptoms of disordered eating, increased body positivity, improved self-esteem, and maintaining a healthy weight.

Cravings versus hunger

There are several methods to distinguish between an actual hunger pang and a yearning.

First of all, keep in mind that while cravings are usually geared toward certain foods or food groups, hunger is a universal emotion.

How to avoid being tempted

Alright, so what steps can you take to reduce your cravings? First, think about the reason for your cravings: an unbalanced diet.

Cravings or Hunger? How to Perceive Hunger Indications

Recognizing your hunger cues is essential to your general well-being, but it's not always simple. Discover how to interpret your body's signals of hunger with these astute techniques. Pay attention to your body. Though it's one of the most frequently given health advice, what does it mean?

It's more difficult than ever to tune out the chatter and pay attention to what our bodies are telling us in a culture that supports restrictive diets and prescribed eating patterns. This is particularly true when it comes to distinguishing between your general health and well-being and hunger cues.

In light of this, let's discuss how to understand and interpret hunger cues to improve the mind-body connection.

What is the meaning of hunger?

Let's begin with the fundamentals: What is the meaning of hunger? Most likely, you are familiar with the emotion. Panting, weariness, and an unquenchable hunger pang. However, did you know that there are two distinct forms of hunger?

Hunger in the body

A physical need to eat is the source of the feeling known as physical hunger. This type of hunger subsides once you eat, and the physical symptoms go away.

Physical indicators of hunger

What signals hunger are? In a nutshell, they're the cues our bodies give us when we're hungry.

There are a few typical hunger cues, however they differ from person to person. How to Tell Whether You're Hungry:

- Growling in the stomach

-Exhaustion or a lack of energy

-Irritability -Shakiness -Dizziness - Nausea -Difficulty Focusing

Hunger on an emotional level

Have you ever questioned why, after eating, you feel hungry?

It's possible that you didn't eat enough, or it could be emotional hunger, which is a desire to eat based on emotions and frequently motivated by what your mouth or mind wants. Sensitive starvation regularly crashes

unaccompanied by caution, satisfaction meals lead to your obsession.

Eating while experiencing a distressing or intense feeling, such as anger, worry, or despair

an incapacity to put food down when full

guilt feelings following a meal

Emotional hunger might also manifest as mindless eating. Guidance on concentrating on one's anatomy.

You can utilize the hunger scale in conjunction with these mindfulness techniques to become more in tune with your body and adopt a more instinctive eating style.

Give yourself a moment. It might only take a few minutes or thirty seconds. Lie your hands on your abdomen and sense what it feels like. Does it feel empty? Does it emit rumbling noises?

What sensations come to mind when you think about food—both inside your body and outside? What level of energy are you at right now?

Become inquisitive. Identify the type of food your body is craving: is it sweet, salty, or savory? How may that hunger be satisfied by a well-balanced meal?

Decelerate. Consume your food mindfully. Give each bite some thought and appreciate it.

Expert advice: To slow down and savor your meal, put your silverware down in between mouthfuls.

Register. Once you've finished eating, take another look at your physique and note your feelings. Did the cuisine meet your expectations? Did it meet your needs? Do you still experience any signs of hunger?

The Emotional Bond with Meal

Enjoying food and eating it is vital to our physical and emotional well-being. Nutrient-dense meals are necessary for our bodies to be nourished and to satiate physical hunger. Nonetheless focusing on meals for sensitive relief, relaxation, or personality benefits is roughly globally acknowledged.

When we do this, we frequently grab harmful options like candy or junk food.

Proportionally on the other hand it may appear like sensitive consumption enhances faith in oneself but doesn't address emotional issues. In actuality, it frequently exacerbates symptoms.

In addition to the initial emotional problem, you might experience guilt for overindulging in food.

Does eating improve our mood?

An emotional hole or a feeling of emptiness can be brought on by negative emotions. Food is viewed physiologically as a means of temporarily satisfying that hunger and producing a false sense of "fullness."

Emotional eating is not uncommon, and there's nothing wrong with treating yourself to food as a treat, reward, or occasion to celebrate now and then.

"Nonetheless, provided that sensitive consumption is your major conscious adaptive process and takes place regularly, this can elevate some red lights."

When the drive to satisfy emotional demands through food takes precedence over or replaces a healthy eating pattern, unhealthy problems result.

Take a look at some of these useful suggestions for improving your connection with food and your lifestyle.

Do I eat based on my emotions?

Although there are many similarities between physical and emotional hunger, there are also important distinctions between the two.

Keep track of when and how you become hungry, as well as how you feel after eating.

An uncontrollable, vital sensitivity is sophisticated, just after being abruptly beaten by sensitive starvation.

In contrast, physical hunger increases more gradually and, unless you haven't eaten in a long time, the need to eat doesn't feel as urgent or require immediate gratification.

 Emotional hunger is more likely to be the cause of a need for a certain food type, such as sweet snacks, candies, chocolate, pizza, fries, etc.

Almost anything, even nutritious food, seems good when you're physically hungry.

Mindless eating is typically the result of emotional hunger.

You don't even notice you've finished a tub of ice cream or a bag of chips because you weren't enjoying them. You are usually more conscious of what you are doing and how much you are eating if you eat because you are physically hungry.

Just after you are substantially satisfied, sensitive starvation goes on insatiable.

On the other hand, you don't have to feel stuffed to feel fulfilled from physical hunger; you might feel satisfied while your stomach is full.

Your belly is not the origin of sensitive starvation.

As opposed to experiencing a knot in your stomach or a rumbling stomach, you "feel" your hunger as an insatiable mental need.

It frequently results in regret, shame, or guilt. You won't likely experience regret or shame when you eat to satiate physical hunger because you are providing your body with what it needs at the moment.

You may realize deep down that you're not eating for nourishment if you feel bad after eating.

Strategies for addressing emotional eating

Look for further stress-reduction strategies.

Many a time, the initial tread on the road to getting control of passionate ingestion is discovering a robust selection for dealing with feelings. Each person has a different solution.

It could involve taking a walk, journaling, reading, playing sports, taking a class, or just finding some time to unwind and unwind from the day. It takes time to change your mindset and routines, participate in a range of healthy stress-relieving activities, and try out different things until you find what suits you best.

What effects do different emotional coping methods have on focus?

Engage in mindfulness. To improve your attitude and adopt healthy habits, try breathing exercises, relaxation techniques, or meditation in a peaceful place.

Keep a food journal. Safeguarding a publication of your refreshments under some circumstances may be of use to you in deciding the characteristics that supply sensitive ingestion. You can use nutrition tracking software or take notes in a notepad.

Try recording everything you eat, no matter how little, and how you're feeling at the time, even if it can be difficult. Your food diary might be an invaluable tool to share with your doctor if you decide to seek medical attention for your eating habits.

Consume a balanced diet. Make sure your body receives the right amount of diverse minerals and vitamins. Eating healthily throughout the day usually makes it simpler to recognize when you're overindulging in food. Consume plenty of water and nutritious food to prevent mindless munching. Take out of your kitchen everything enticing high-fat, high-calorie, or sweet meals and junk food. Furthermore, do not go grocery shopping while you are irritated or hungry.

Be mindful of serving sizes. To help with portion management, measure out servings and use tiny plates; with time, these mindful eating practices will become second nature. Give yourself some time after consuming a serving size before returning for another, and sip lots of water in between.

Get help from those you love. Speak with a close friend or member of your family if you're feeling depressed, anxious, or alone to help lift your spirits. Formal support groups are another valuable resource. Finally, if you feel lost or powerless, ask your physician for advice and a recommendation to a coach or counselor who may assist you in pinpointing the emotions causing your hunger pangs. Disorganized Consumption is undoubtedly a solemn indisposition that can be generated by sensitive ingestion. Taking care of the emotions underlying the habit is critical to long-term wellness. Every day, approach the process with a new perspective. This helps you become a better version of yourself and cultivate healthier eating and eating-related relationships with food.

Chapter 2: Identifying Unhealthy Eating Patterns

Common Diet Pitfalls
1. Eliminating favored meals.

It's difficult to stick to a diet when you can never eat your favorite foods. Suddenly, those foods seem especially attractive, and before you realize it, you're "cheating" on your diet and feeling defeated. Allowing yourself to indulge once in a while (savoring those meals without feeling guilty) can help you find a healthy balance that works long-term.

2: Eliminating whole types of meals

There's a reason carbs, fats, and protein are called macronutrients: your body requires them in massive amounts. A diet plan that urges you to eliminate any of these main groups may cause problems in the long run.

For example, the fat-phobic 1990s gave rise to a variety of sugary refined carbs, and Americans acquired massive amounts of weight.

3. Expecting too much too soon.

Many doctors think that healthy, long-term weight loss should be limited to one to two pounds per week. If you expect to lose weight faster than that, you may become discouraged. But slow and steady wins the race, so stick with it!

4: Skipping meals.

Skipping meals may appear to be a great way to save calories, but it might lead to overeating later on. If you skip lunch, for example, you may overeat at dinner, believing that the extra calories are justified. Eat when you're hungry (but not ravenous) to keep hunger and portion sizes under control.

5: Eating too little.

If you want to lose weight quickly, it may be tempting to cut calories drastically but proceed with caution. Diets with too few calories do not provide all of the nutrients your body needs.

Make 1,200 calories your minimum daily calorie goal. With proper planning, you can consume a balanced diet for that amount.

6: Eating because the plan says so.

On the other hand, if your plan requires you to eat every two or three hours but you are not hungry, that is not necessarily a good thing.

To maintain a healthy weight, you must learn to recognize and respond to your internal hunger cues; therefore, if you're hungry, eat; if you're not, don't.

7: Thinking exercise allows you to pass.

When striving to reduce weight, exercise, and dieting must be combined; however, the goal is to increase exercise (calorie burn) while decreasing calorie intake. It's easy to overestimate how much you burned during an exercise session and then overeat to compensate, which defeats the purpose. Stick to the rule of thumb that unless you exercise for an hour or longer, you only need water to replenish your body afterward.

The Power of Habit

Understanding the power of habit can help you spot unhealthy eating patterns and make beneficial changes. Habits are repetitive acts that we engage in without much conscious thought, and they can be extremely effective in shaping our diets.

Knowing how habits work allows us to identify problematic ones and develop strategies to replace them with healthier alternatives.

Here are some important factors to consider while examining the strength of unhealthy eating habits:

Habitual Cues: Our environment and habits frequently stimulate specific eating tendencies. These cues could be anything from the time of day, the people we're with, to the sight of specific meals. Identifying these warning indicators is critical since it allows you to predict and avoid risky decisions.

Automatic Behaviors: When a cue is triggered, habitual behavior occurs almost automatically.

This can include mindless snacking while watching TV, grabbing quick food when you're pressed for time, or finishing everything on your plate even if you're already full. Recognizing these natural responses is crucial to breaking the pattern.

Variable incentives promote habits, and food can be an effective reward. However, the benefits of improper eating are typically fleeting and may have serious long-term consequences. Identifying the genuine rewards you seek (comfort, convenience, social connection) will help you find healthier ways to meet those needs.

Ideas and Expectations: Our beliefs and expectations about food and ourselves can influence our eating habits.

For example, if you think nutritious food is bland and unappealing, you'll be less inclined to stick with it. Challenging these limiting beliefs and creating a more positive association with healthy eating can be motivating.

Plans for Change: Once you've discovered your unhealthy eating habits, you'll need to devise change strategies.

This may involve:

Swapping sugary drinks for water, keeping nutritious snacks on hand, or planning your meals ahead of time will help you avoid harmful temptations.

Becoming mindful of your eating: Pay attention to your hunger and fullness cues, eat slowly, and taste your food.

Experiment with healthy alternatives: Look for nutritious recipes that are both delicious and fulfilling.

Looking for assistance: get in touch with an authorized dietician or psychiatrist for customized reinforcement. Remember that changing behaviors requires time and effort. Be patient with yourself, appreciate your accomplishments, and don't be discouraged by setbacks.

By recognizing the power of habit and implementing these strategies, you may regain control of your eating habits and make positive changes for a healthier you.

Identifying Emotional Eating Triggers

Emotional eating is the act of consuming food based on feelings and emotions rather than hunger or nutritional needs. It can be produced by a variety of emotions, including anxiety, boredom, depression, or even happiness. Sensitive ingestion regularly contributes to greed and the absorption of harmful nourishment, one and the other may subsidize fattening up and harm

Universal well-being.

Sensitive consumption is an ordinary adapting mechanism for responding to agony and pessimist sensitization. Humans often get involved with nourishment for consolation, as it supplies short-term relief of their sorrow.

Unfortunately, short-term satisfaction can have long-term negative consequences for both physical and mental health.

In this post, we will look at the emotional eating cycle, the distinction between emotional and physical hunger, how to identify your triggers and effective ways to reduce emotional eating.

Emotional Eating

Sensitive consumption patterns consist of a chronology of incidents and reactions that strengthen the practice of consuming concerning emotions. This cycle frequently follows a pattern.

psychological cause: an incident or feeling, like nervousness or hopelessness, gives rise to Consumption for solace or deviation.

The sensitive catalyst leads to the shooting up of starvation.

Overeating: The individual indulges in comfort eating, consuming more food than is necessary to satisfy hunger.

Guilt and shame: Following overeating, feelings of guilt and shame arise, which can further worsen the emotional distress.

Reciprocate: whenever a moving sensitive generation develops, the pattern kicks off, and the passionate consumption habit proceeds.

Smashing the poignant consumption pattern compels recognizing and working out basic emotions and prompts, together with executing suitable adaptive mechanisms.

Emotional hunger versus physical hunger.

Understanding the distinction between emotional and physical hunger is essential for overcoming emotional eating and maintaining a healthy diet.

Recognizing these contrasts can allow you to respond appropriately to your body's requirements and avoid overeating or eating unhealthy foods for emotional comfort.

These are the visible things for both:

Onset: Emotional hunger typically appears abruptly and seems urgent, prompting you to eat immediately. Physical hunger, on the other hand, develops gradually, giving you time to decide when and what to eat, and can be delayed without creating anxiety.

Desires: Emotional hunger frequently results in cravings for specific comfort foods, such as sweet, fatty, or high-calorie treats. Physical hunger, on the other hand, is more adaptable and can be satisfied with a variety of food options.

Saturation: sensitive starvation is not fulfilled when you are filled, which may bring on greediness. Natural craving vanishes after taking sufficient dietary to retain your anatomy

functioning, showing that it is a moment to quit feasting.

Culinary behavior: sensitive consumption is differentiated by fast, thoughtless, expanding, and deficient pleasure in ingestion exposure.

In contrast, eating to satisfy physical hunger is often a more conscious and satisfying experience, with emphasis on the flavor and texture of the meal.

Sensitive outcome: sensitive consumption humiliates you from the people around you. In contrast, eating to satisfy physical hunger has no emotional burden because it is a natural response to your body's needs for food and energy.

Emotional hunger manifests itself as a craving in your mind rather than a sensation in your stomach. Physical hunger, on the other hand, is typically sensed as stomach rumbling or slight discomfort, indicating the need to eat.

Triggers: Emotional hunger is typically triggered by specific sensations or situations, such as stress, boredom, or grief, whereas physical hunger is caused by the body's demand for nourishment following a period of fasting.

Recognizing these differences is critical for overcoming emotional eating since it helps you become more aware of your body's true needs and avoid using food as a coping mechanism for emotions.

Distinguishing between emotional and physical hunger motivates you to make healthier choices, eat a more balanced diet, and have a better connection with food.

Uncover Your Emotional Eating Triggers: Path to Self-Awareness Anxious-woman-eating

Sensitive feasting prompts are incidences, scenes, or feelings that result in ingestion for reasoning other than starvation or sustenance.

By recognizing these triggers and why eating can imply finding, you can start to end the pattern of sensitive ingestion. Common emotional eating triggers include:

Stress: When your stress levels rise, your body produces cortisol, a hormone that can cause an increase in hunger. Eating comfort foods may temporarily relieve stress, resulting in a cycle of emotional eating.

Boredom: In the absence of stimulation, boredom may drive you to seek excitement or distraction through food, particularly overeating or indulging in unhealthy meals.

Infant habits: Eating habits formed during infancy may persist throughout maturity.

For example, if you were given food as a reward for good behavior or achievement, you may associate eating with comfort and validation, leading to emotional eating in response to feelings of inadequacy or low self-worth.

Social situations: Parties, parties, or eating out with friends may encourage overindulgence or comfort food. Popular belief or the urgency to suit it may also lead to sensitive consumption.

Negative emotions: Sadness, loneliness, fury, or frustration can drive people to seek solace in food, using it as a temporary escape from their emotional pain. Consuming high-calorie, sugary, or fatty foods may provide a brief sense of relief, but this usually leads to overeating and perpetuates the cycle of emotional eating.

To recognize your sensitive consumption catalysts, retain a nourishment publication.

This technique comprises taking notes on what you eat when you eat, and the feelings or circumstances surrounding each episode of emotional eating.

Eventually, logic order will become evident, disclosing the precise catalysts that produce your sensitive consumption incidents.

How To Stop Emotional Eating

Practice mindfulness and mindful eating.

Mindfulness is the practice of being fully present and aware of one's thoughts, emotions, and physical sensations. Incorporating mindfulness into your eating habits may help you detect Emotional hunger and avoid overeating.

Mindful eating practices include eating deliberately, savoring each bite, and focusing on the flavor and texture of the meal. To incorporate mindfulness into your daily life, try meditation or deep-breathing exercises, and make a concerted effort to concentrate on your dining experiences.

Develop alternative coping skills.

Boost your managing power for responding to agony and unacceptable sensations rather than consuming sensitively. For example, physical activity can reduce stress and improve mood by releasing endorphins.

Consider blogging, talking to a friend, or using relaxation techniques such as deep breathing or progressive muscle relaxation.

Experiment with several coping skills to see which ones work best for you.

Create a support network.

Cherishing a backing system could be accommodative in conquering sensitive ingestion, get in touch with comrades or in-laws who are aware of your strives and can encourage, assist, and are liable to you.

Keep a food and mood diary.

As told earlier, preserving nourishment and emotional publication may assist you in recognizing sensitive consumption causes and arrangements. Monitoring what you eat, when you eat, and the emotions or situations that promote emotional eating will provide you with valuable insights into your relationship with food. Utilize this data to advance anthropomorphize plans of carrying on with your prompts and beating sensitive consumption. There are a variety of software and tools available to assist you in successfully tracking your eating habits and emotions.

Develop a healthy environment.

Making changes to your environment may significantly impact your eating habits.

Keep tempting, hazardous foods out of reach, and instead stock your kitchen with nutritious, wholesome options.

Dishing up a blooming bite to eat in advance will ease the ability to select nourishment when sensitive starvation hits. Additionally, create designated dining areas in your home to reduce mindless nibbling in front of the TV or computer.

Set reasonable goals and enjoy small triumphs.

Changing the course of sensitive ingestion demands schedule and commitment.

Set reasonable and manageable goals for yourself, and celebrate small victories along the way.

For example, if you successfully manage your emotions without using food, recognize your achievement and reward yourself with a non-food indulgence, such as a relaxing bath or a new book. Positive reinforcement can boost your confidence in your ability to overcome emotional eating.

Be patient and kind to yourself.

Remember that overcoming emotional eating is a gradual process with potential setbacks.

It's critical to practice self-compassion and patience with yourself as you attempt to develop good eating habits. In case you blunder, acknowledge the fact, become proficient in it, and proceed.

Expanding a sort of advanced knowledge in connection with

yourself can outstandingly boost your universal health and victory in abstaining from sensitive ingestion. service guidelines.

Your assessment may comprise nourishment handling protocols, policies, potential it(administrative evaluation), and distinct particulars and drinks provided.

Evaluation of Food Service Policies, Practices, and Capacity

You can use a tool like the food service guidelines evaluation tool to examine food service policies, procedures, and capability in your preferred site. To complete the assessment, ask members of your team who are familiar with your agency's food procurement and preparation practices. However, the questions will differ based on the needs of your agency.

Usually, these include:

-Type of company and the number of employees or customers.

-Food service establishments that prepare, serve, and sell food.

-The rules, norms, and practices that govern food purchasing and nutrition.

-The extent of your jurisdiction over what foods are sold.

-The contracting process and processes for purchasing goods and food services.
-The ability to apply food service guidelines.
Nutrition
Search Menu
Navigation Menu
Nutrition
Build a foundation.

Assess the food environment.

Conducting a baseline assessment of the food environment is crucial for determining where adjustments are required and what resources will be beneficial. It will also allow you to track progress after you have created food service guidelines. Your evaluation could include food service regulations, practices, capabilities (organizational assessment), and specific items and beverages offered.
Evaluation of Food Service Policies, Practices, and Capacity.

Restaurant host

You can utilize an assessment tool, such as
Food Service Guidelines Organizational.Assessment, to

gather information about food service policies, procedures, and capability in your preferred setting. To complete the assessment, ask members of your team who are familiar with your agency's food procurement and preparation practices.

The questions will vary depending on the needs of your agency, but generally include:

-Type of company and the number of employees or customers.

-Food service establishments that prepare, serve, and sell food.

-The rules, norms, and practices that govern food purchasing and nutrition.

-The extent of your jurisdiction over what foods are sold.

-The contracting process and processes for purchasing goods and food services.

-The ability to apply food service guidelines. **Evaluation of certain foods and beverages**

Before you begin establishing food service laws, determine how well the food and beverages served in your establishments adhere to these criteria. This information provides a baseline for:

- Determine what percentage of goods and beverages presently meet specific food and nutrition standards outlined in the guidelines.

-Establish goals for executing the nourishment handling protocols that can be withstood progressively.

-Use frequent measures to track changes over time and enhance the program.

Maintain compliance with food service requirements.

Chapter 3. The Science Behind Cravings and Hunger

It is crucial to perform a baseline assessment of the food environment to identify areas that require development and identify valuable resources. In addition, tracking adjustments will be possible after the implementation of food service guidelines. Your evaluation may encompass aspects such as food service policies, procedures, capacity, and the particular cuisines and beverages provided.

Critical Analysis of Food Service Capabilities, Policies, and Practices

In the setting of your choosing, you may utilize an assessment instrument such as the food service guidelines assessment tool to evaluate food service policies, practices, and capacity. Collaborate with team members who possess knowledge of the food procurement and preparation procedures of your organization to accomplish the evaluation.

In general, the inquiries may differ contingent upon the specific requirements of your agency; however, they typically comprise the following: -Number of employees or patrons and nature of the organization.

-Appointments for food service in which food is sold, prepared, or served.

-Prevalent policies, standards, and practices that have an impact on the procurement of food and nutritional aspects.

-Scope of your authority over what commodities are sold.

-Contracting process and procedures for purchasing foods and food services.

-Capacity to implement culinary service guidelines.

-Nutrition

-Search Menu -Navigation Menu - Nutrition

-Build a foundation

Assess Food Environment

It is crucial to perform a baseline assessment of the food environment to identify areas that require development and identify valuable resources.

In addition, tracking adjustments will be possible after the implementation of food service guidelines. Your evaluation comprises nourishment aid guidelines and distinct sustenance and drinks provided.

Restaurant host

You can use an assessment instrument such as the Food Service Guidelines Organizational Assessment instrument pdf to collect information about food service policies, practices, and capacity in your setting of choice.

Collaborate with team members who possess knowledge of the food procurement and preparation procedures of your organization to accomplish the evaluation. The questions will vary depending on the requirements of your agency, but generally they include:

-categorization of corporations and the number of workers or sponsors.

-Nourishment protocols are destinations where nourishment is made ready, dished out, or vented.

-Current directives, criteria, and routines that influence the purchase of foodstuffs and nourishment.

Scope of your authority over what commodities are sold.

-Contracting process and procedures for purchasing foods and food services.

-Capacity to implement culinary service guidelines.

Assessment of Specific Foods and Beverages

Before you begin using food service guidelines, ascertain the extent to which food and beverages offered in your settings meet these guidelines. This information provides a baseline for:

Determine what percentage of foods and beverages already satisfy specific food and nutrition standards in the guidelines.

Inaugurate policies for executing the nourishment certification requirements that can be relevant in supplementary hours.

Track changes over time with repeated measurements for program enhancement.

Monitor compliance with food service guidelines.

The Physiology of Hunger and Satiety

Lack of food fullness sequence necessitates ante-consumption and Hippocratic and Synaptic procedures. Consuming, one after the other triggers preventive signs to generate gratification.

Imperceptible

From the perspective presented in this minireview, it is evident that a variety of psychological and physiological factors interact to regulate feeding behavior. Due to the delay between the ingestion of food and the breaking down of cuisine, the sufficiency procedure calls for a temporary indicator to curb greediness. This temporal Saturation sign is energized by mental influence, compound feelings, and automatic features associated with the procedure of consumption and gastrocolic inflation. The excellent management of eating conduct through these procedures will guarantee the conservation of ordinary power consumption.

It is crucial to note, however, that despite all the efforts that have gone into the study of peripheral and central mechanisms of ingestive behavior--expressed in thousands of publications associated with the physical, attractiveness and digestion, biology, and habitual features of consuming. we will lack an understanding of the interactions among signals within a system or among distinct systems.

Why We Crave Unhealthy Foods
Here are some key reasons: Brain's Reward System:

Pleasure chemicals: Unhealthy foods are often packed with sugar, salt, and fat, which stimulate the release of dopamine and other "feel-good" chemicals in the brain. This creates a pleasurable experience that reinforces the desire to consume more of that substance.

Evolutionary holdover: From an evolutionary standpoint, these high-calorie nutrients were once scarce and essential for survival.

Our minds are wired to seek out such foods, even if they are no longer necessary for survival in our modern environment.

Hormonal Influences
Stress hormones: When agitated, our bodies produce

cortisol, which can increase appetite and cravings for sugary or fatty foods. This is a temporary coping mechanism but can become problematic if stress is chronic.

Hormonal fluctuations: Hormonal changes during the menstrual cycle or pregnancy can also contribute to cravings for specific foods.

Other Factors:

Dehydration: Sometimes, thirst can be misinterpreted as appetite, leading to cravings for sugary or salty snacks instead of water.

Habit and emotional eating: Comfort foods associated with positive memories or used to cope with negative emotions can induce cravings, even if they are unhealthy.

Marketing and accessibility: Unhealthy foods are often heavily marketed and readily available, making it simpler to choose them over healthier options.

It's important to remember that cravings are not a sign of weakness, but rather a complex response to numerous internal and external factors. Understanding the triggers can help you develop strategies to manage them and make healthier choices. Here are some tips:

Identify your triggers: Pay attention to what situations or emotions contribute to cravings for unhealthy foods.

Plan wholesome alternatives: Have healthy snacks readily available to satiate cravings without indulging in unhealthy options.

Practice self-compassion: Don't beat yourself up if you give in to a yearning. Just attempt to get back on track with your healthy eating goals.

Remember, implementing sustainable changes takes time and effort. Put up with yourself and commemorate your advancement in transit.

Debunking food misconceptions

We are regularly compelled on what to consume and what not to from different publications. Unfortunately, not all this advice is accurate, and many nutrition fallacies persist despite scientific evidence to the contrary.

Here are 10 common nutrition misconceptions we'll debunk to help you

**make informed choices
about your diet.
Being obese makes you
obese**

The belief that eating fat makes you acquire weight has been debunked. Healthy lipids, such as those found in avocados, nuts, olive oil, and fish are essential for your body's functions. Including these in small amounts does not contribute to weight gain. Too much calorie consumption, regardless of the essential nutrients they contain, can subsidize fattening.

All calories are comparable

Some calories are what we term "empty calories". This shows that they give us more or less nourishment excluding vigor. Nutrient-dense foods like vegetables and lean proteins provide more nutritional value than empty-calorie garbage foods.

Consuming late hours may contribute to fattening.

The hour you consume is less important than the stand of nourishment you partake. As long as your "energy in equals energy out", eating late at night won't inherently contribute to weight gain.

What matters most is the content of your late-night nibble and the overall daily energy intake.

Detox regimens are necessary

Detox diets and cleanses often promise to remove impurities from your body, but your body has its detoxification systems in place.

Instead of detox diets, concentrate on eating a balanced diet rich in whole grains (fiber), fruits, and vegetables (antioxidants) to support your body's natural detoxification processes. This will also help to keep your gut bacteria content.

All protein sources are comparable

While protein is essential for creating and repairing tissues, not all protein sources are equal. Animal-based proteins such as lean meats and fish, eggs, and dairy foods are known as complete proteins, meaning they contain all the essential amino acids necessary to construct and repair tissues. Plant-based proteins like legumes and lentils (except soybeans) are not complete proteins, meaning they lack one or two of the essential amino acids. Soy (tofu, edamame, tempeh) is a complete protein and makes an excellent choice for vegetarians and vegans. Combining different grains and legumes can also create complete proteins.

Skipping meals assists with weight loss

Skipping meals can slow down your metabolism and contribute to overeating later in the day.

It's better to consume regular, balanced meals and snacks to maintain steady energy levels and control your appetite.

Egg yolks are harmful to your cholesterol

For years, egg yolks were demonized due to their cholesterol content. However, recent research has shown that dietary cholesterol has a minimal impact on blood cholesterol levels for most individuals. Eggs are a nutrient-rich food that can be part of a healthful diet.

All sugar is the same

There are various types of sugar in the foods we eat. Fruits have natural sugars that come with fiber and essential nutrients, but processed foods have added sugars that have little nutritional value. Your health needs to limit the quantity of added sugars you consume.

You need to consume meat to get enough protein

While meat is an excellent source of complete proteins, you can get all the protein you need from a vegetarian or vegan diet by incorporating tofu products and by including a variety of beans, peas, lentils, nuts, seeds, and whole grains. A balanced plant-based diet can provide ample complete protein – you just need to make sure that you're consuming a combination of these foods.

Nutrition is a complex and ever-evolving field, and misinformation can make it challenging to make healthful choices. By debunking these 10 common nutrition myths, we aim to empower you to make informed decisions about your diet. Remember that a balanced and varied diet, rich in whole foods, is essential to maintaining good health.

Part 2: Breaking the Cycle: Unlearning Bad Habits
Chapter 4: Mindfulness and mindful eating

The Power of Present Moment Awareness

Mindfulness, the practice of focusing on the present moment without judgment, holds immense power, especially when applied to our relationship with food. This practice, translated into mindful eating, empowers us to cultivate a healthier and more fulfilling connection with nourishment. Let's delve into the transformative potential of moment awareness in mindful eating.

Breaking the autopilot: We often eat on autopilot, driven by distractions and external cues. Moment awareness disrupts this automatic mode, urging us to be present with our food and internal signals.

By tuning into physical sensations like hunger, fullness, and taste, we regain control over our eating choices.

Mindful Cues, not Calorie Counting: Instead of obsessing over numbers on a scale, mindful eating focuses on internal cues. We learn to distinguish true hunger from emotional triggers like stress or boredom.

This shift empowers us to make conscious decisions about what, when, and how much to eat, fostering a healthier relationship with food.

Savor the Senses: Moment awareness awakens our senses, transforming meals into mindful experiences. We appreciate the colors, textures, and aromas of each bite, allowing us to truly savor the flavor and enjoy the process of eating. This mindful appreciation fosters gratitude and satisfaction, reducing the urge to overeat.

Non-judgmental Approach: Mindful eating encourages self-compassion and non-judgment towards our eating habits and choices. We acknowledge, without criticism, the thoughts and emotions that arise during meals, leading to a more peaceful and accepting relationship with food.

Stress reduction and emotional regulation: The present-moment focus of mindful eating helps us manage stress and regulate emotions, two common triggers for unhealthy eating patterns. By becoming aware of our emotional state, we can make conscious choices about whether or not to eat and what to choose, reducing stress-induced eating.

Improved digestion and overall well-being: Mindful eating promotes slower, more intentional chewing, aiding in proper digestion and nutrient absorption. The reduced stress and emotional eating also contribute to improved overall well-being and a healthy gut microbiome.

Remember: The strength of mindful eating rests in its simplicity.

By increasing moment awareness with each bite, we uncover a transforming journey towards a healthier and more joyful relationship with food. It's not about perfection, but about intentionally engaging with the present moment and choosing choices that nourish our body and mind.

Mindfulness, the practice of focusing on the present moment without judgment, carries great power, especially when applied to our relationship with food. This practice, translated into mindful eating, helps us to create a healthier and more rewarding connection with sustenance. Let's look into the transforming power of moment awareness in mindful eating.

Breaking the Autopilot: We often eat on autopilot, influenced by distractions and external stimuli. Moment awareness breaks this automatic phase, forcing us to be present with our food and internal cues. By tuning into physical feelings like hunger, fullness, and taste, we recover control over our food decisions.

Mindful Clues, not Calorie Counting: Instead of stressing over numbers on a scale, mindful eating focuses on internal clues.

We learn to separate actual hunger from emotional causes like stress or boredom. This transformation empowers us to make intentional decisions about what, when, and how much to consume, promoting a healthy relationship with food.

Savor the Senses: Moment awareness wakes our senses, transforming meals into mindful experiences. We appreciate the colors, textures, and scents of each bite, allowing us to genuinely savor the flavor and enjoy the process of eating. This focused appreciation generates gratitude and satisfaction, lessening the need to overeat.

Non-judgmental Approach: Mindful eating supports self-compassion and non-judgment towards our eating habits and decisions. We notice, without condemnation, the thoughts and emotions that come during meals, leading to a more calm and accepting connection with food.

Stress Reduction and Emotional Regulation: The present-moment concentration of mindful eating helps us manage stress and regulate emotions, two major triggers for harmful eating patterns.

By becoming aware of our emotional state, we may make conscious decisions about whether or not to eat and what to choose, lowering stress-induced eating.

Advanced ingestion and universal health: careful consumption motivates steady, organized dining, reinforcing visual metabolism and nourishing consumption. The lowered stress and emotional eating also contribute to enhanced general well-being and a healthy gut microbiota.

Remember: The strength of mindful eating rests in its simplicity. By increasing moment awareness with each bite, we uncover a transforming journey towards a healthier and more joyful relationship with food. It's not about perfection, but about intentionally engaging with the present moment and choosing choices that nourish our body and mind.

Cultivating Mindful Eating Practices

Eating as thoughtfully as we do on retreat or in mindfulness training is not possible for many of us, especially with families, careers, and the countless distractions around us. This is not to say that our comrades, in-laws, and co-workers can not have the tolerance to consume with us even though we may take about five minutes to take our bites.

So have a little self-recognition, and take a look at approved observant consumption on resorts and significant moments, in addition to casual knowledgeable metabolism in your systematic existence.

What is Mindful Eating?

Mindful eating, or mindful eating, is the practice of being fully attentive to your food, your feelings, your hunger, and your satiety indicators. It's about eating deliberately, engaging all senses, and noting responses, sensations, and physical signs like hunger or fullness.

Incorporating mindful eating habits into our daily routine isn't simply about eating slower or choosing nutritious meals; it's about fostering a more intimate and intentional relationship with what we consume. By learning how to eat slower and more deliberately, we can not only enjoy our meals more but also become better attuned to our body's requirements, leading to enhanced well-being and happiness.

6 Ways to Practice Mindful Eating

Cautious consumption helps in making fresh nourishment selections and putting up practices that improve both somatic and psychological well-being. Here are six mindful eating ideas to get started eating more mindfully:

1) Allow your anatomy to come to your intellect

Eating swiftly past full and rejecting your body's signals vs. slowing down and stopping when your body indicates it's full.

Slowing down is one of the finest ways we can get our minds and bodies to express what we need for nutrition. Our anatomy neurotransmitters communicate a score before our cerebellum and this is the reason we are over scorched accidentally. But, if we slow down, you can give your body a chance to catch up to your brain and hear the messages. Easy methods to decelerate comprise noting countless of your granny practices, as well as easing off to ingest, biting each nourishment 25 times, placing your fork down between bites, and all those ancient manners that are maybe not as pointless as they looked.

Food for thought: What are a few different ways you can dial back consumption and pay attention to your embodiment signs?

2) Know your body's particular hunger signals

Frequently we concentrate first on our leads, but like many knowledgeable methods, we could locate significant understanding by converting to our embodiments first.

Rather than just eating when we get emotional signals, which may be different for each of us, whether they stress, unhappiness, irritation, loneliness, or even plain boredom, we can listen to our body. Is your stomach growling, energy low, or feeling a touch lightheaded? Too frequently, we eat when our head tells us to, rather than our bodies. True mindful eating involves genuinely listening deeply to our body's signals for hunger.

Speculate: What are your anatomy's starvation signs, and what are your psychological ravenousness causes?

3) Nature a solicitous cookery for knowledgeable consumption
Eating alone and randomly vs. eating with others at established times and places.

Differently, we eat thoughtlessly by loitering around checking into closets, consuming aimlessly at any time, preferably fairly reasoning cautiously regarding our nourishments and refreshments. This decelerates us in one way but stops us from growing well ecological prompts about the quantity and what we eat, and twists our mental capacity for modern prompts of consumption that are not perfect at all times.

Certainly, we all consume refreshments once in a while, this may improve your brain and embodiment well-being which gradually assists your emotional state rest scheme to consume at compatible hours. Yes, that includes sitting down, putting food on a plate or dish, not eating it out of the container, and using utensils, not our hands.

You don't have to plan your diet down to each bite, and it's vital to be flexible, especially during special events, but simply be aware of the fact that you might be modifying your eating patterns at different times of the year or for different occasions. In addition to organizing, you are also probably going to eat the amount your body requires at that moment rather than undereating and indulging later, or overdoing and regretting it later.

The classic recommendation is to also not shop when hungry, but the middle route applies here as well. A psychological phenomenon known as "moral licensing" has demonstrated that buyers who buy kale are more likely to then head to the booze or ice cream aisle than those who don't. We seem to conceptualize that our feelings will compensate and we might "squander" them on processed food, or other subordinate-absolute measures.

4) Understand your motivations

Eating foods that are emotionally soothing vs. eating nutritionally beneficial things.

This is another tough balance, and ideally, we can choose nourishing foods that are also tasty and comfortable.

But think back to that first conscious raisin. Did that look appealing before you tried it? There are numerous rationale the consumption of dried grapes is such an influential effort, nevertheless one is that when we slow down and eat good things like raisins, we often enjoy them more than the tale we tell ourselves about healthy meals. As we practice eating better and a broader range of meals, we are less prone to binge on our comfort foods, and more inclined to appreciate healthy foods, ultimately finding many foods psychologically and physically rewarding as opposed to just a few.

5) Connect more closely with your food

Considering where food comes from vs. Reasoning of consumption as a finished outcome.

Unless you are a hunter-gatherer or sustenance farmer, we have all become even more detached from our food in recent years.

Many of us don't even realize where a meal originates from outside the shop packaging.

This is a loss because eating offers a great opportunity to link us more intimately to the natural world, the elements, and to one another.

When we cease to reckon all of the individuals associated with the nourishments that has come on your plate, from the loved ones (and yourself) who prepared it to those who supplied the racks, to those who sowed and gathered In the fresh components, to those who supported them, it is hard not to feel both grateful and interconnected.

Be cognizant of the water, land, and other factors that were part of its formation as you settle down to eat whatever you are eating. You can ponder on the cultural traditions that brought you this meal, the recipes kindly given by friends or brought from a distant place and time to be handed down in the family.

When giving thought to every single thing that happened in the nourishment, it enhances easiness to familiarize with and convey thankfulness to all of the humans who committed their hours and strive, the constituents of the cosmos that triggered their share ration, our allies or forefathers who split methods and also the individuals who might have disposed their existence to a part of creating this meal.

With just a little more attention like this, we may begin to make wiser choices regarding sustainability and health in our food, not only for us but for the whole planet.

6) Attend to your plate Distracted eating vs. mindful eating.

Multifunctioning and consumption is a method for not being able to pay attention to our embodiment's requirements and desires. We've all had the experience of going to the movies with our bag full of popcorn, and before the coming attractions are done, we are inquiring who ate all of our popcorn. When we are preoccupied, it becomes tougher to listen to our body's cues regarding food and other demands. With your succeeding nourishment, attempt sole-tasking and fair consumption, with no displays or interference apart from loving the comrades you are having nourishment and conversation with.

So while formal mindful eating practices may be what we think about when we look back on a mindfulness training or retreat we attended, the truth is that we live, and eat, in the real world, which is a busy place.

Nevertheless, we can take some understanding acquired from our official operation - decelerate, pay attention to your embodiment doing one thing in a moment, expanding corresponding minor ways, and bearing in mind everything that occurred in our refreshments on an increased systematic ground, ushering in further casual knowledge to our day-to-day nourishments.

Using Mindfulness to Manage Cravings

Food cravings may be a tremendous force, often leading to unwise decisions and harming our well-being. But the good news is that mindfulness may be a great technique to help us manage them in a healthy and lasting way. Here are some crucial practices:

1. Acknowledge and Observe:

Don't judge: When a hunger arises, resist the urge to categorize it as "good" or "bad." Simply notice it as a sensation in your body, like a wave in the ocean.
Notice the details: Pay attention to where you sense the need and its strength. Is it sharp or dull? Pulsating or constant?

2. Detach and Label:

Observe your thoughts: Notice any stories or judgments related to the craving.
Recognize them as thoughts, not facts.
Label the need: Give it a name, such as "sugar craving" or "boredom craving." This helps create space between you and the urge.

3. Explore Alternatives:

Ask yourself: Do you need to eat right now, or is there another need driving the craving?

Engage in self-care: Consider other strategies to meet your underlying need, such as drinking water, taking a stroll, or stretching.

4. Mindful Eating:

If you choose to eat: Do so mindfully. Savor each bite, and observe the taste, texture, and aroma. Slow down and eat until comfortably full, not stuffed.

Additional Tips:

Practice regularly: Mindfulness is a skill that grows with practice.
Start with short meditation sessions and integrate thoughtful moments throughout your day.
Be patient: Don't expect perfection. There will be times when cravings triumph, but each conscious moment is a step forward.
Seek support: Consider attending a mindfulness group or working with a therapist specializing in mindful eating.

Chapter 5: Building a Balanced Plate Understanding

Macronutrients and Micronutrients

These essential elements from fats, protein, carbs, vitamins, and minerals help your body work properly.

What are macronutrients?

As the main nutrients found in food, macronutrients support your body's structure and functioning.
You usually need a large amount of macronutrients to keep your body working properly. But don't stress: macronutrients come from proteins, fats, and carbs, which give your body energy in the form of calories. Macros are usually measured in grams (g) and can be a useful way to track what you're consuming.
Overall, counting macros is a way to focus on the range of foods you're eating — and how much of each — instead of counting calories.

Examples of macronutrients

Throughout metabolism, nourishments that seem to come in one of the three supplements are digested to be used for diverse motives. Macronutrients include:

Carbohydrates.

As the main source of energy, carbs break down into glucose and help digestion and fullness. Carbs include bread, rice, pasta, grains, fruits, starchy veggies, beans, milk and yogurt. They provide 4 calories per gram.

Fat: is broken down into fatty acids and glycerol and provides fat-soluble vitamins A, D, E, and K.

Protein: helps build and repair muscle, tissues, and organs, as well as aid in hormone control. Foods like meat, chicken, fish, eggs, cheese, cottage cheese, plain Greek yogurt, and tofu provide 4 calories per gram.

Examples of vitamins

Just like macronutrients, micronutrients can be found in the foods that you eat every day — think fruits and veggies.

Some vitamins that are examples of minerals include:.

Vitamin C. Also known as ascorbic acid, vitamin C is needed for the creation of neurotransmitters and collagen. Minerals that are ideal for supplements include:

Calcium. This mineral helps build strong bones and teeth and helps with muscle performance.

Magnesium. Found in foods like pumpkin seeds, almonds, and spinach, this mineral aids in the control of blood pressure.

Sodium. You need sodium for optimal fluid balance and to keep your blood pressure.

Potassium. Potassium helps with muscle movement and nerve transmission. You can find potassium in foods like peaches, lentils, prunes, and raisins.

Why are macronutrients and vitamins important?

They are the nutritive constituents required by the body in large quantities for our body's well-being.

Creating Nutritious and Delicious Meals

Creating nutritious and delicious meals is doable! It can be fun, too, with the right attitude.

These are some things we need to take note of:

Planning and Prep:

Balance is key: Aim for a healthy plate with each meal, including:

Half non-starchy vegetables: Think bright veggies like broccoli, carrots, bell peppers, leafy greens, etc.

Quarter lean protein: Choose lean meats, fish, fowl, legumes, tofu, or eggs.

Quarter whole grains: Opt for brown rice, quinoa, whole-wheat pasta, or other whole grains.

Meal planning: This saves time and money. Plan your meals for the week, considering dietary restrictions and tastes.

Prepping ingredients: Washing, chopping, and storing veggies or marinating protein beforehand simplifies cooking later.

Cooking Techniques:

Seasoning is your friend: Experiment with herbs, spices, and flavorful ingredients to add depth without counting on unhealthy additives.

Healthy cooking methods: Use grilling, baking, steaming, or stir-frying instead of frying to keep nutrients and reduce fat.

Small changes, big impact: Swap white rice for brown, use lean ground turkey instead of beef, or add spinach to your pasta sauce.

Recipe Resources:

Explore online recipe websites and cookbooks: Look for ones dedicated to healthy and delicious meals.

Utilize cooking apps: Many offer recipe ideas, meal-planning tools, and grocery lists.

Consider food restrictions: Find recipes that can cater to vegetarian, vegan, gluten-free, or other needs.

Additional Tips:

Get creative: Don't be afraid to play with flavors and ingredients.

Make it visual: Colorful and well-presented meals are more appealing.

Involve others: Cooking with family or friends can be fun and informative.

Don't strive for perfection: Enjoy the process and celebrate your wins!

Portion Control and Mindful Eating

Our eating habits have changed dramatically in recent times with the abundance of ready-to-eat foods in the market which are lip-smacking and tasty.

Moreover our progressively fast-moving way of living, we have begun to eat greedily fast foods from vendors/ street cafes for convenience.

This is happening sometimes purely due to lack of time but a lot of times due to easy access to these foods and snacks. It is hard to avoid such foods in our everyday lifestyle, but what is possible is to understand how we can moderate the consumption of such processed foods by practicing portion control in our daily meals.

There are plenty of studies on how large portion sizes can have an impact on health.

To effect change, the key is to change the way we snack and eat our everyday meals carefully keeping portion sizes in mind.

In addition to this, it is important to understand and implement ways we can replace junk and unhealthy foods with healthier snacking choices.

Understanding Mindful Eating

When babies are given birth they are well known for eating only while hungry.

But as we grow up, we tend to be exposed to a lot more food, fad diets, irregular meal times, work pressure, worry, lack of exercise, and a whole lot more.

These changes to our lives incite us to overeat, thereby making us unable to stop eating when we are full and in turn throw the entire cycle of eating into a tailspin.

When we consistently overeat, even if it's healthy food, it tends to leave us feeling a bit tired, and sluggish, and finally over time throws our body weight and health off the charts.

When it comes to keeping good health, losing weight, or even fighting lifestyle-linked diseases like diabetes, hypertension, high cholesterol, and more - maintaining and eating the right portion sizes which includes, adding the right food groups to our diet plays a key role.

Portion control along with careful eating is one of the core essences of good nutrition, apart from the micro & macro nutrients we add to our diet. It is not about losing weight or watching calories. It is a healthy habit we can adopt to develop a positive relationship we have with our food and our body.

What are the guidelines needed when portioning

A share is the quantity of nourishment you fill in your platter; it is the quantity of refreshment required for your embodiment's satisfaction. It is not easy to quantify the amount of nourishment partaken, nevertheless, there are effortless ways to determine if you are consuming the correct quantity.

One of the keys to thoughtful eating is to eat the right foods when you are hungry and stop when your mind says it's full or is getting full. Hence it is vital to pay attention to your amount size when watching your diet. In addition, paying attention to your portion size and eating a balanced meal will give your gut enough time to send the signal to the brain that you are satiated and are getting full.

To get a feel for how much carbs, protein, fats, and veggies to have in a meal, use the plate or a palm rule to measure out amounts.

The following are guidelines on diverse ways of consuming knowledgeably with the right measurement our embodiments require.

Making your food healthy is about using the right cooking methods, the right ingredients, and cooking with fresh seasonal ingredients. In addition, we need to limit the consumption of pre-processed foods for eating as well as during the process of cooking.

In most cases, we fail to consider fine nourishments in our daily refreshments. A great way to think of planning a menu for a meal is by cooking a range of dishes and adding colors to your plate.

Your plate should look bright and include food from the various food groups. This ensures your body is getting proper nutrition.

Once you have included the right food groups in your meal, you must exercise portion control so you don't overeat. One of the ways we can ensure we can incorporate the right portion sizes is by using measures that are practical and something we can continue.

For example, using slotted thali plates or using categories helps us measure the amounts of the food.

The slotted plates also ensure that you cook a variety of meals for as many slots/ cavities as are there in the slotted plate. Slotted plates also ensure that you eat only what you have given yourself on the plate.

The following are some categories of meals you can consider when preparing nourishment.

Protein

Proteins are important building blocks that help the body build and repair tissue, muscles, cartilage, and skin, as well as pump blood. Most

Indians fail to meet their daily protein needs in their everyday diet. Research says that about 30% of your daily diet should consist of protein.

Proteins can be in the form of whole dals, paneer, tofu, chana, rajma, milk, dahi, green veggies, eggs, sprouts, chicken, or fish.

Therefore, having one helping of protein-based dishes with every meal is important for maintaining good health. Bodybuilding assists you extensively, as your embodiment sticks around in breaking down them.

Having adequate protein during your meals slows down the digestion process and helps us feel more full and less likely to get a quick bout of hunger pangs during the day.

Fats

There are good fats and bad fats and most often people tend to avoid any fatty food.

As a general concept, it is a good thing, but our body does require a certain amount of fats, and here's why. Dietary fats are important to give your body energy and to support cell growth. Fats help protect your organs and are important for the body as they synthesize hormones, store vitamins and provide energy.

Research says that your diet must consist of healthy fats – polyunsaturated, monounsaturated, and Omega-3 fatty acids.

Using restricted amounts of ghee, mustard oil, coconut oil, sesame oil, groundnut oil, sunflower oil or even rice bran oil is the most optimal way to consume fats. In addition, there are many things we already eat - milk, curd, eggs, chicken, and fish; all of them also contain good fats that are important for our diet.

What is important to remember is to avoid deep-fried foods and highly processed foods which contain a lot of trans fat. Many a time, it is necessary to employ rationing the quantity of fine and harmful paunchy we consume. If the puree is well, this is not enough reason to make us abide by a casein diet and consume beyond what our body can hold.

If fats are fine for us, that does not signify we prepare and consume only fat-rich nourishments. Eating all fats in the right amounts is extremely important.

That amount is something you can determine based on your body type, your requirement for health, and suggestions given by your nutritionist or doctor.

Carbohydrates

Energy-giving foods are vital for the embodiment, as it is one of the major Genesis of energy.

It is paramount to select and consume the good type of carbohydrates.

Avoid carb-rich processed foods like bread and biscuits which are also known to be simple carbs. When making rotis, and parathas, make your atta multigrain by adding flours like ragi flour, jowar flour, and bajra flour which are whole-grain flours that contain complex carbohydrates.

If you are a rice eater then opt for brown rice or millets which have more fiber and protein. If you are making dosa batter, then add millets like ragi, bajra, and jowar to improve your fiber content.

Adding fiber-rich carbohydrates, packed with nutrients also known as complex carbs to the diet helps slow the eating process and keeps you feeling full for longer.

Vitamins & Minerals & Fibre

Vitamins and minerals especially Vitamin A, E, B12, D, Calcium, and Iron are important for the body. Vitamins and Minerals help in better metabolism, muscle function, bone health, and cell production.

It's important to include a good amount of fruits, vegetables, green leafy vegetables, colorful salads, nuts, and dry fruits throughout the day either in your meal or during the mid-morning

snacks or the evening snack.

Include a lot of raw veggies in the form of salads in at least two meals. Indian salads are great because they are simple and quick to make and can be made tasty and chatpata with locally available ingredients.

Adding raw vegetables and fruits to your diet will also ensure you get the proper fiber your body needs to stay healthy.

Eat Slowly

Eating slowly is often forgotten when we are sitting for a meal with family at a table or when we are having lunch at the office or even at a restaurant. When there is a lot of food kept on a table, or when there is a lot of work on our mind, we tend to eat fast and in the process miss maintaining portion amounts.

Research has shown that it takes 12 or more minutes for food satisfaction cues to reach the brain.

Consuming without hurrying can help you have adequate hours for better communication between the gut brain and the main brain.

The perks of slow eating can bring a lot of health to our lives and is one of the simplest things we can practice. Chewing well and eating slowly helps in better metabolism. Eating slowly, also helps us be careful about our portion sizes which helps in weight loss or weight maintenance.

On the other hand, eating quickly leads to bad digestion, increased weight gain, and lower levels of satisfaction that we have eaten enough.

Take precautions on the nourishments you consume

Being mindful is an exercise that is very important to practice in today's times. Our lives are fast-paced and packed with different activities and duties we need to perform during the day. During this process, we tend to forget the most important parts of our day - which are meal and snack times. We tend to pay less attention to it and try to pack in tasks that keep our minds stimulated with everything else but food.

Here is where being careful about the food you eat comes in, which can help you lead a healthy lifestyle.

A great way to be careful about what goes into your body is to keep mobile phones, TV, books, newspapers, and miscellaneous distractions out of your sight or the dinner table.

If you are at home, with the family, ensure that you have a well laid out table with plates and spoons, and food is put out on the table in small serving bowls.

These small tips help bring awareness to what you eat and how much you eat. Your attention is on your food and the time you spend with your family. You are aware of what you consume and what you put into your platter and your embodiment.

If you are at work at your desk, then closing your laptop and keeping your phone turned face-down will help you focus on the food in your lunch box.

Having the least amount of distractions helps us focus on the food we eat, helps us be in the moment with family, friends, and workers, and most importantly helps us eat portion-controlled meals.

Chapter 6: Emotional Eating Management.

We don't always consume just to gratify somatic starvation. Many of us turn to food for comfort, stress relief, or to treat ourselves. When we do, we tend to go for junk food, candy, and other comforting but unhealthy options. Sensitive eating is the use of nutrients to revitalize yourself—to fill your psychological desires rather than your stomach. Sadly, sensitivity consumption does not sort out sensitive subjects. It frequently makes you feel bad. Not only does the initial emotional issue remain, but you also feel terrible about consuming.

Are you an emotional eater? Do you overeat when you're stressed?

Do you eat to feel better (to soothe and console yourself when you're upset, annoyed, bored, anxious, etc.)? Do you reward yourself with food? Do you usually eat until you're stuffed? Do foods make you feel safe? Do you ever feel helpless or out of control around food? A sensitive consumption pattern of frequently using nourishments as an energizer, a present, or to make clear isn't automatically a pessimist thing.

But if nourishment is your main sensitive managing way —when your first feeling is to navigate the freezer whenever you're nervous, troubled, sad, isolated, worn out, or disinterested —you're confined in an unhealthy cycle in which the real sensation or problem is never addressed. Emotional hunger cannot be satisfied by food. Eating may appear pleasurable at the time, yet the feelings that prompted the eating persist. And you frequently feel worse than you did before because of the unnecessary energy you've just consumed. You blame yourself for making mistakes and lacking willpower.

Compounding the problem, you stop learning new ways to deal with your emotions, you have a more difficult time controlling your weight, and you feel increasingly powerless over both food and your emotions. Regardless of how powerless you feel over food and your emotions, it is possible to make a positive change. You can learn healthy strategies to deal with your emotions, avoid triggers, overcome cravings, and finally end emotional eating. The difference between emotional and physical hunger. Before terminating the way of sensitive consumption, you must acknowledge the contrast between sensitive and somatic starvation. This may be more difficult than it appears, especially if you frequently use food to cope with your troubles. Emotional hunger can be intense, making it easy to confuse it with physical hunger. However, some signs might help you tell the difference between physical and emotional hunger. Emotional hunger arises suddenly. It strikes you immediately and seems stunning and critical. Physical hunger, on the other hand, develops more gradually. The desire to eat is less intense and does not require immediate gratification. Emotional hunger craves specific comfort foods. When you're physically hungry, almost everything sounds good—even nutritious foods like vegetables. Nevertheless sensitive starvation longs for processed nourishments or sappy refreshments that supply an instant high. You desire cheesecake or pizza, and naught will be sufficient. Emotional hunger often results in mindless eating. Before you know it, you've finished an entire bag of chips or a pint of ice cream without paying attention or fully enjoying it. When you eat in response to physical hunger, you are usually more conscious of what you are doing. Emotional hunger is not satisfied once you're full. You remain craving increasingly, consuming until you're intolerable. Physical hunger, on the other hand, does not have to be satisfied. You feel content when your belly is filled. Emotional hunger is not located in the stomach. Rather than a growling belly or an ache in your stomach, you experience hunger as a persistent need that cannot be satisfied. You concentrate on specific textures, tastes, and scents. Emotional hunger frequently results in regret, shame, or humiliation.

When you eat to satisfy physical hunger, you are unlikely to feel guilty or humiliated because you are merely providing for your body's requirements. If you feel bad after eating, it's probably because you realize you're not eating for nutrition. Find your emotional eating triggers. The first step in overcoming emotional eating is to understand your triggers. What situations, places, or emotions cause you to seek the comfort of food? Most emotional eating is associated with negative emotions, but it can also be induced by positive emotions, such as rewarding yourself for achieving a goal or celebrating a holiday or celebratory occasion. Common causes of emotional eating: Stress. Have you ever noticed how stress makes you hungry? It's not only in your mind. When stress is persistent, as it often is in our hectic, fast-paced world, your body produces large amounts of the stress hormone cortisol. Cortisol stimulates cravings for salty, sweet, and fried foods—foods that provide a rush of energy and satisfaction. The more unmanageable pressure in your existence, the more possible you are to involve yourself in nourishment for sensitive support. Stuffing feelings.

Consumption can be used for a time to subdue or "consume " pessimist feelings like antagonism, agitation, sorrow, nervousness, isolation, bitterness, and humiliation. While you're anesthetizing yourself with refreshments, you can disregard the hard feelings you'd preferably abstain. Boredom or a sense of emptiness. Do you ever eat just to have something to do, to relieve boredom, or to fill a void in your life? You feel unfulfilled and empty, and eating serves as a means of filling your mouth and occupying your time. simultaneously, it saturates and diverts you from your fundamental emotions of uselessness and discontentment with living.

Childhood habits. Think back on your childhood eating experiences. Did your parents reward good behavior with ice cream, take you out for pizza after you received a good report card, or feed you sweets when you were sad? These habits can often persist until maturity. Or your eating habits may be motivated by nostalgia—fond memories of grilling burgers in the garden with your father or baking and munching cookies with your mother.

Social influences. Meeting up with others for a meal is a great way to relieve tension, but it can also lead to overeating. It's easy to overeat just because the food is accessible or everyone else is eating. You may also gluttonize in social circumstances due to nervousness. Perhaps your family or circle of friends encourages you to eat too much, and it's easy to follow suit. Maintain an emotional eating diary. You've probably recognized yourself in at least a couple of the preceding descriptions. Even so, you'll want to be even more specific. Keeping a food and mood journal is one of the best ways to identify the themes that underpin your emotional eating habits. When you binge or feel coerced to seize your version of solace refreshments, vulnerability , take a little while to contemplate what activated the desire. If you go back, you'll usually find an upsetting event that sets off the emotional eating cycle. Write everything down in your food and mood diary: what you ate, what disturbed you, how you felt before eating, how you felt while eating, and how you felt afterward. Over time, you will notice a pattern emerge.

In most cases, we gluttonize when spending time with colleagues or when in in-laws' conventions. Once you've identified your emotional eating triggers, the next step is to find healthier ways to feed your feelings. Find new ways to nourish your feelings. If you cannot find a way to do away with your emotions, it will be after controlling your craving desires in the future.Diets frequently fail because they provide acceptable nutritional advice that is only effective if you maintain conscious control over your eating habits. It fails when emotions take over the process, expecting an immediate reward in the form of food. To quit emotional eating, you must find new ways to satisfy yourself emotionally.

Comprehending the rotation of sensitive consumption, or even acknowledging your catalyst, is not enough, nevertheless, it is a vital beginning. You require alternative sources of emotional fulfillment besides eating. If you're nervous, channel your energy by dancing to your favorite song, squeezing a stress ball, or taking a quick stroll. If you're tired, make yourself a hot cup of tea, take a bath, light some scented candles, or wrap yourself in a cozy blanket.

If you're bored, try reading a good book, watching a comedy program, going outside, or doing anything you enjoy. Halt when hunger attacks, and check in with yourself. The predominance of sensitive consumers trust that they have out of the hand of their hunger. When the need to eat arises, it is all you can think about. You sense an almost unbearable tension that has to be fed right now! Because you've already attempted to resist and failed, you believe your willpower isn't strong enough. But the truth is that you have more control over your cravings than you think. But if you can pause and reflect when you're faced with hunger, you give yourself the option to make a better choice. Can you delay eating for five minutes? Or simply start with one minute. Don't tell yourself you can't give in to hunger; remember that the restriction is quite attractive. Simply convince yourself to wait. While you wait, check in with yourself. How do you feel? What is going on emotionally? Even if you do eat, you'll have a better understanding of why you did so. This can help you prepare for a different answer the following time. Learn to accept your feelings, including the negative ones.

Though the main problem may be a deficiency over refreshments, sensitive consumption stems from a sense of incompetence over one's feelings. You don't feel capable of confronting your emotions head-on, so you avoid them with food. Allowing yourself to experience uncomfortable emotions can be difficult. But the truth is that when we don't concentrate on or hide our emotions, even the most painful and difficult sentiments fade quickly and lose their ability to direct our attention. To accomplish this, you must practice mindfulness and learn to stay tuned to your current emotional experience. This can assist you in doing away with tension and convey sensitive matters that regularly contribute to sensitive consumption. Support yourself with healthy lifestyle choices. When you're physically strong, relaxed, and rested, you're better prepared to deal with the unexpected challenges that life throws at you. However, when you're already exhausted and overburdened, each minor malfunction can drive you off track and straight to the refrigerator. Make daily exercise a priority. Physical activity improves your mood and energy levels while also helping to reduce stress. And getting into the workout habit is easier than you would think. Purpose not less than eight hours of rest per night. When you don't get enough sleep, your body craves sugary meals that give you a quick energy boost. Getting plenty of rest might help with appetite control and reduce food cravings. Make time for pleasure. Allow yourself at least 30 minutes per day to relax, decompress, and unwind. This is your opportunity to take a break from your responsibilities and recharge. Connect with others. Do not underestimate the value of close connections and social activities. Spending time with wonderful people who brighten your life will help you avoid the negative effects of stress.

Chapter 7: Meal Planning and Preparation

When it comes to maintaining a healthy lifestyle, conserving time, and successfully managing finances, meal planning and preparation are essential components.

Several actions and considerations need to be taken to guarantee that meals are nourishing, well-balanced, and pleasurable. A comprehensive approach to the

planning and preparation of meals is as follows:
Determine the dietary requirements and preferences:
You and your family members should take into consideration any dietary restrictions, allergies, or health goals that you may have.
Make sure that you take note of your food preferences and dislikes so that you can enjoy your meals.
Create a menu for the week by:
You should make a plan for the upcoming week's meals, which should include breakfast, lunch, dinner, and snacks.
At each meal, you should strive to consume an appropriate amount of fruits, vegetables, healthy fats, carbohydrates, and proteins.
If you want to avoid boredom and make sure you are getting a wide range of nutrients, include variation.

Make a shopping list:

Based on the planned meals, develop a detailed shopping list of the ingredients needed.
Check your pantry and fridge for products you already have to avoid wasteful purchases.
Choose Recipes:

Select dishes that correspond with your menu plan and dietary limitations.

Look for recipes that are quick to make, or try batch cooking for efficiency.

Consider meal prep techniques:

Batch cooking: Prepare large quantities of staple foods like grains, meats, and vegetables to utilize throughout the week.

Pre-cut and wash fruits and vegetables to save time during meal preparation.

Utilize slow cookers, pressure cookers, or one-pot recipes for convenient cooking.

Set aside time for preparation:

Choose a certain day or time each week for meal planning and preparation.

Allocate sufficient time to cook, portion, and store meals for the week ahead.

Storage and Portion Control:

Invest in excellent storage containers that are appropriate for refrigerating or freezing meals.

Portion meals appropriately to avoid overeating and to streamline meal distribution throughout the week.

Healthy Swaps and Modifications:

Experiment with healthier alternatives to standard ingredients to increase nutrition (e.g., using whole grains instead of refined grains, and substituting lean meats for fatty ones).

Reduce additional sugars, salt, and bad fats in dishes without compromising flavor.

Consider Convenience Foods Wisely:

While convenience foods might save time, seek out healthier products with minimal additives and preservatives.

Use pre-cut vegetables, canned beans, or frozen fruits as shortcuts for meal preparation.

Review and adapt:Regularly examine your meal plan and preparation process to identify areas for improvement.

Adjust portion sizes, recipes, or meal frequency depending on comments and changing nutritional needs.

Chapter 8: Building a Supportive Environment

Building a supportive atmosphere is vital for various facets of life, from personal well-being to the performance of teams and organizations. Enlisting the help of others plays a vital part in creating this supportive climate. Here's how:

Understanding the Need for Help:

Recognize that no one individual can be everything to everyone. Reaching out for and accepting aid is a sign of strength, not weakness. Identify places where further support is needed. This could be emotional, physical, logistical, or even simply having someone to listen to.

Identifying Potential Helpers:

Consider your network: friends, family, colleagues, neighbors, community groups, or faith-based institutions.
Look for persons with relevant talents, experiences, or resources that correspond with your needs.

Consider professional support networks like therapists, counselors, or coaches.

Asking for Help Effectively:

Be precise about your needs. The more information you share, the easier it is for others to offer relevant support.

Communicate your expectations and boundaries. What sort of help are you looking for? How much time or participation are you comfortable with?

Express gratitude for their willingness to help, even if they can't supply exactly what you need.

Building Collaborative Relationships:

Remember, assistance is a two-way street. Be open to giving support to others in return when you can.

Foster open communication and respect throughout your support network.

Celebrate triumphs and offer encouragement through adversity.

Be cognizant of power dynamics and ensure everyone feels heard and appreciated.

Additional Tips:

Leverage internet resources and support groups suited to your requirements or scenario.

Consider joining workshops or programs focused on fostering supportive environments.

Don't be scared to distribute jobs or share responsibility.

Remember: Asking for help is a critical step in developing a supportive atmosphere. By finding prospective helpers, communicating effectively, and creating collaborative relationships, you may create a network that empowers you and people around you.

Creating a Healthy Home Food Environment
Clear Your Home of Less-healthy Food

These foods are okay in moderation, but they may be eaten outside of the house pleasantly and powerfully.

Go through your kitchen fridge, freezer, pantry, cabinets and counters to discard out goods that aren't helping you accomplish your health goals.

Put Healthy Foods in Plain Sight

Keep grab-n-go fruit on the counter instead of snack foods so they are conveniently available. Consider placing your perishable fruit on a shelf at eye level instead of keeping it in the crisper. Vice versa, transfer less healthy foods to the crisper so they aren't always in your line of sight.

Find Healthy Substitutions

Feeling deprived of your favorite foods might make you unpleasant and bitter. Instead, experiment with healthier choices. Here are several examples:

Calorie-controlled frozen yogurt bars vs high-calorie ice cream novelties

Sparkling water versus soda or fruit juice

Skinny popcorn vs chips and crackers

Clean and Organize

A dirty kitchen might make it challenging to find healthy choices when you are hungry or short on time. It is also difficult to find

whatever you require from the food
mart. Give your kitchen a New
Year makeover and organize your
food storage places so you can
always locate what you need
without distraction.

Eat at Your Kitchen Table

Eating at your kitchen table without
interruptions is a way to eat more
consciously and enjoy time with
your family.

Eating on the couch while watching
shows or movies can encourage
thoughtless eating and absorbing
more calories than intended.

Keep Healthy Foods Readily Available

When you are hungry and in a
pinch, it's crucial to have nutritious
items on hand so you don't make
hunger-controlled choices. This
includes keeping ready-to-go snack
foods in your kitchen such as fruit
paired with nut butter, hummus,
and carrots, lunch meat and cheese
roll-ups, etc. It may also assist in
keeping prepackaged freezer
dinners on hand for hectic

weeknights when you don't have
time to make supper.

Managing Social Eating Situations

Navigating social eating doesn't have to be as tough as it may now feel. With a few basic social eating tips that you can keep in mind, it will seem much easier for you to exercise balance with your meal choices.

Set a Clear Intention

In addition to being mindful, you can also develop a clear goal of what you'd like to experience during the event or gathering.

Are you there to catch up with old friends you haven't seen in a while? To jubilate the matrimony of two of your in-laws? To enjoy the great food at your favorite restaurant?

Or maybe you want to be able to eat food at an event without constraint or guilt so you can focus on mingling and not get caught up in food rules.

These are all objectives where physical nourishment isn't the primary priority – and that's OK! Sometimes enjoyment is the priority instead.

If that's the case, allow yourself to actively appreciate the setting and what you're there to experience, rather than obsessing on food restrictions or the "shoulds" that you can think of.

When you're no longer at the social gathering and back into your routines, nourishment can become more of a focus again. This is the balance we teach within the Method that allows you to ebb and flow between sustenance and enjoyment throughout the numerous phases of your life.

Build Balanced Meals and Snacks

The best way to keep stability in collective consumption situations is to flashback the dogma of evened consumption practices. One of the key techniques we teach our customers is how to make a balanced meal or snack.This helps kids to get the nourishment they need while also enjoying the foods they love, no matter where they are!

We do this utilizing our Foundational Five system, and if you're not familiar with this system yet, you can download our free Balanced Eating Guide that lays out exactly what to include on your plate for balance. Keeping this simple system in mind during social gatherings will make it so much less stressful for you. You'll be able to look at any buffet, charcuterie board, or snack table and be able to simply imagine what you can add to your plate to create a balanced meal.

Will your meals from the buffet look like the meals you create at home, probably not, but again – that's OK!

The Foundational Five framework gives you the direction you need to know that you're doing your best in every given setting, so you can approach any social encounter with confidence.

Bring a Nourishing Option to Share

With that being said, knowing that most social events have a lot of pleasurable foods but tend to lack nutritional foods, is there something you might bring to share that is both nourishing and enjoyable?

Stay Mindful

It might be easy to get caught up in the moment at social events, especially with that shift of environment and peer pressure we just talked about.

One method we provide with our Mindful Nutrition Method™ members to assist them combat this is to be mindful in social situations.

What exactly do we mean by mindful? Well, let's say your aunt is pushing you to eat her brownies, or maybe you're strolling by a dessert table with all kinds of sweets and delights.

And let's assume you don't like brownies, or sweets aren't really your thing, but in the past, you almost always would just grab a handful of anything off of the sweets table because it was simply there, or say yes to the brownies just because she insisted.

Does this ring sound familiar to anyone? These are examples of thoughtless eating, which is a key contributor to the lack of balance you've felt in social situations in the past.

This time, put mindfulness into play. If you are aware that what she is offering you is not your preference , talk with yourself. Do you genuinely want the brownie?

If not, simply say no thank you. If you know you're more of a savory person rather than sweet, keep on going by that table and spend your time elsewhere where it's delightful for you.

Having mindfulness in these moments will allow you to make decisions that feel truly good and right to you, which will assist you to eliminate that sense of tension, guilt, or overwhelm that occurs as a result of imbalanced eating in social eating situations.

Practice Balance the Day of your Social Event

Now there will also be circumstances where you're not able to bring a nourishing option, or you simply may not want to. Such as if you're heading out to eat at a restaurant or to your parents' place for your mom's legendary trifle.

In those cases, you might focus on exercising balance not only during the social function but also throughout the entire day.

If you know you're going to be experiencing food products that are predominantly on the enjoyment end of the Balance Spectrum, you can prioritize some nourishing food items at other points during the day.

Now we're not talking about fasting the day off, or "making up for" the enjoyment of food thereafter, because we know those aren't examples of balanced eating habits. We're merely talking about establishing a balance between nourishment and fun rather than falling to all-or-nothing thinking.

If you're going out for a birthday dinner and know the alternatives are all enjoyment foods, you can focus on getting a nutrient-dense smoothie and a veggie-packed bowl for lunch so your body has what it needs to feel fantastic.But don't let this produce worry — remember that this isn't black and white, it's about big-picture thinking. It's about establishing overall equilibrium.

Prepare to Communicate Your Boundaries

Peer pressure is very widespread during social events and we hear from many clients who feel the need to eat in the same way as others or feel pressured by relatives and friends who are remarking on what they are or are not eating. Unfortunately, you're likely to experience this at some time in your path.

Having a couple of sentences in mind that you can use can be beneficial for setting your boundaries and ending the conversation.

Chapter 9: Transitions to a Sustainable Lifestyle

Creating Achievable and Realistic Goals
Give specifics: specify precise objectives

When defining goals, be as detailed as you can and be as exact as you can. Only when you have clear objectives can you know what you are aiming for? Establishing specific goals has the benefit of allowing for quantifiable success.

Let's say you wish to construct a home. Normally you will try to construct the most pretty building. What do you think "pretty" means? How many rooms ought to be there? If so, what size garden should there be? The same applies to your personal and professional objectives: The more precise they are, the more effectively you can organize and proceed.

It also gives you a better overview of your present progress by making goals measurable.

Defining and detailing your objectives might also help you feel more motivated. It supports your ability to maintain concentration and move toward your goal with reasonable measures.

Keep it real: Please, don't go overboard.

It's tempting to set high standards for yourself. However, ambition frequently equates to false expectations. Unrealistic ambitions can have a detrimental effect on success: Frustration and self-doubt mount if you fail to accomplish any of them.

For instance, it is usually unrealistic to set goals like learning a new language flawlessly in a month.

This objective may swiftly demoralize you to the point where you want to give up.

Such lofty objectives require a great deal of patience and time to accomplish. Alternatively, you may aim for the following goal: "I will be able to introduce myself in the new language I have learned and respond to inquiries about my work in less than a month."

Being realistic does not imply a lack of ambition; on the contrary, long-term success is reserved for those who accurately assess their capabilities! Even with increased complexity and difficulty, goals still need to be reachable.

Additionally, it has been demonstrated that establishing goals linked to performance might boost intrinsic motivation. I'll get to my next point now.

Ask yourself a question: What drives you personally?

Recognize why you desire to accomplish a particular goal.

This is also known as intrinsic motivation, which is the desire to accomplish goals based on your motivation. Higher levels of internalized and intrinsic motivation are linked to improved job performance and a higher sense of well-being.

Does this imply that managers should stop defining goals for their staff members and instead allow individuals to set their own? I wouldn't quite agree with that; in light of the previously mentioned factors, you ought to try establishing objectives that your staff finds appealing. Together with your staff, establish goals and involve them in the decision-making process.

It is encouraging to work for organizations where employees from many nations collaborate.

After all, our intrinsic motivation is influenced by both our cultural background and our individual ability level.

As a manager, you should always be inquisitive and mindful of the motivations and preferences of your staff.

Be devoted: Share your objectives with everyone.

Informing your loved ones, friends, or coworkers about your aim increases your chances of success. This boosts motivation and fosters commitment.

Establish benchmarks: Establish checkpoints along the route.

While deadlines are necessary for goals, long-term goals also require milestones. They can serve as significant interim goals or checkpoints, for instance, after project phases, allowing you to assess if your plan is still working as intended. The team or supervisor can, at most, have a once-over look at them if the goal appears to be very well-served.

Milestones boost motivation by demonstrating your advancement. If you always feel like you are stagnating and not getting anywhere, it can be incredibly discouraging. Even celebrate a tiny victory to maintain your motivation! Going back to the foreign language example: You may make a weekly commitment to learning ten new terms.

Your intermediate objective can be to place food orders in the local tongue when you go on your next vacation to a particular nation.

These modest objectives assist you in maintaining motivation as well as in recognizing and resolving issues before they worsen.

Sustaining Motivation Over Time

To ensure that lifestyle modifications are sustained, persistence is essential. While the initial thrill will help you get through the beginning, longer-term commitment calls for more sophisticated tactics.

Obstacles to Sustaining Motivation:

Routines & Habits: Because we are creatures of habit, it can be difficult to break long-standing habits. New habits may seem unique at first, but old patterns may reappear.

Setbacks & Plateaus: Not all progress is linear. Setbacks and plateaus can be demoralizing, resulting in a decline in motivation and possibly a relapse.

Lifestyle Friction: New routines can be difficult to maintain and can be disrupted by outside circumstances such as social gatherings, travel, or professional pressures.

Long-Term Motivation Techniques:

Put Intrinsic Rewards First: Link your adjustments to your objectives and core beliefs rather than merely to outside influences. What aspects of this shift are really important to you?

Establish wise objectives: Goals that are Time-bound, Relevant, Measurable, and Specific give you a sense of progress and defined objectives.

Honor minor victories: Celebrate every accomplishment, no matter how tiny. This helps you feel good about yourself and keeps you going.

Locate a Partner for Accountability: Talk about your aspirations and challenges with an encouraging friend, relative, or online group. Their support and common experience might be quite beneficial.

Exercise self-compassion by forgiving yourself for mistakes and failures. Consider the lessons learned, not setbacks.

Make it Pleasurable: Look for methods to enjoy your new way of life. To make things interesting, try out various games, recipes, or strategies.

Put Progress First Rather Than Perfection: Pursue advancement over perfection. Over time, even tiny, consistent actions result in significant changes.

Visualize Success: Take some time to see yourself accomplishing your objectives and leading the life you have always wanted. Your dedication and motivation may increase as a result.

Seek Support: If you need assistance, don't be afraid to contact a professional. Nutritionists, coaches, and therapists can offer specialized advice and assistance.

Conclusion

"The Starvation Inclination" is not a typical calorie-counting book that focuses only on "ending" eating. Instep, it leaps even higher, exploring the mental and physical mechanisms underlying compulsive eating. Manufacturer Judson Brewer opposes the notion that humans eat habitually due to energy impulses and desire rather than actual starvation.

The main goal of the book is to give people the power to change how they relate to food and their bodies.

It provides a useful foundation for caring for people and changing their eating habits, enabling them to break free from unhealthy eating habits and develop a more thoughtful and responsible approach to eating. Put differently, "The Starvation Propensity" does not provide a magic bullet or an unaffordable diet.

Instep provides a method for navigating change by identifying the primary triggers of binge eating and cultivating a more meaningful connection with food.

The principal ideas

Rather than verified starvation, energetic eating is motivated by inclination and compensatory cues. Comprehending the neurology of desires helps empower people to make informed choices.

To break depressing eating plans, care and affinity modification treatments are essential.

The objective is to promote a more cautious and altered connection with food rather than to "stop" eating.

Generally speaking, keep in mind a succinct framework.

The book itself provides a far deeper analysis of these concepts and provides personalized philosophies based on specific needs.